The Health Wonders of Oil Pulling Therapy

The Ayurvedic Oral Cleansing Practice is the Next Big Thing!

Disclaimer

Contents

Introduction to Oil Pulling –Traditional Method and a New Approach

"A new truth is a new sense, for with it comes the ability to see things we could not see before – and things which cannot be seen by those who do not have the new truth" ~Weston A. Price

Before we jump to the details, let us first find out what is oil pulling all about. Well, oil pulling (also known as oil swishing) is an old remedy where you hold or swish oil in your mouth.

What is Oil Pulling?

Is it that simple? Indeed! People claim that with the help of this simple oil pulling procedure, they got their life back. When you initially introduce the method to somebody and give them details about the benefits of oil pulling, it will be a little difficult for them to believe it. And why not, something as simple as swishing oil in your mouth can hold such great benefits is indeed news that will shock you. However, the results are indeed wonderful and astonishing.

In a nutshell, oil pulling is an ancient Ayurvedic practice for rejuvenation and detox where you take a tablespoon of oil in your mouth and swish it around for a set amount of time and then simply spit it. The procedure is tried and tested and people literally gushed over how their sinus problem, dental health, and allergies were healed and improved. There were even claims of improvement in skin breakout, hormone imbalances, headaches, arthritis, among others. These benefits will be further discussed on in the chapters to come.

Back to oil pulling, old school oil swishers conventionally used virgin sunflower oil or sesame oil for great oil pulling results. Other than that, coconut oil gained popularity as it soon became one of the best options to be used for oil pulling. Coconut oil gained the mainstream position because of the natural qualities the oil possesses itself, including enzymatic, anti-inflammatory, and antimicrobial properties.

The added benefit of using coconut oil for oil pulling is that it also kills the unwanted bacteria that could be hiding in your mouth – the gateway of your entire body. All in all, coconut oil is considered a better option since the taste is much better than the other options.

The Traditional Usage of Oil Pulling

As mentioned earlier, the practice of oil pulling is traditional. Practitioners used the method, as there were claims that it is capable of improving systemic and oral health. This includes improving and healing conditions like migraines, headaches, asthma, diabetes mellitus, as well as skin problems such as acne. Other than that, traditional usage of oil pulling was also practices because it is known as a natural teeth whitener.

The promoters of this practice claim that the procedure of swishing oil in the mouth helps pull out toxins, which are more commonly known as 'ama' in the language of Ayurvedic medicine. Thus, offering great results in reducing inflammation.

The practice, however, received only a little study. There is little evidence to support the claims that were made by the advocates of the unique technique. According to a small study, sesame oil when swished in the mouth is declared as effective at reducing oral bacteria load as well plaque. On the other hand, it didn't stand as effective as an antiseptic mouthwash (chlorhexidine). The concept has been reintroduced now because traditionally it died due to lack of scientific verification and investigation. It was declared by the National Center for

Health Research that, 'It is still unclear whether or how the practice actually works to get rid of bad bacteria in our mouths. It is also unknown what the long term effects on oral and overall health may be.'

Fortunately, the concept was reintroduced with significant scientific support this time.

Current Usage of Traditional Ayurvedic Oral Cleansing Practice

The idea behind oil swishing or oil pulling and its usage today gained popularity during the 1990s. The idea was reintroduced and popularized by one of the early advocates and adopters of the technique, Tummala Koteswara Rao from Bangalor, South India. Koteswara effectively evangelized the concept of oil pulling as a traditional and effective Ayurvedic practice.

Koteswara Rao claimed to various benefits associated with oil pulling since he has experienced them all himself. He also claims to be introduced with the concept through a paper published to All Ukrainian Association of the Academy of Science of the USSR by Fedor Karach. In the paper he advocated the method of oil pulling. He further disclosed that the paper was widely circulated after it was published in German Magazines in the Natur und Medizin (Nature and Medicine) and Natur & Heilen (Nature & Healing). It was further claimed that the same paper persuaded several people around Germanys to practice oil pulling with sunflower oil for more than a century.

With the support of scientific research and extensive promotion as an effective Ayurvedic practice, the practice is currently enjoying great commercial interest and popularity. While sesame oil was traditionally used for the practice of oil pulling, recently various celebrities endorsed the technique with coconut oil, making it the more popular ingredient in the Western world.

How Does Oil Pulling Works?

Now that you are familiar with the practice of oil pulling, let's dig the topic deeper and find out how this unique practice that claims amazing health benefit really works. Keep reading!

What Experimenters and Experts Have to Say

The best way to learn a new technique is to learn it through what the experts and the experimenters have to say.

The American Dental Association reports that there aren't enough scientific studies and evidences available to prove that the method really works wonders in improving oral health or to be recommended as a professional practice. However, when you ask the experimenters, they have a complete different view of it.

While there are no claims that a regular oil pulling practice should replace the traditional oral care at home or regular dental visits, the benefits associated with this popular Ayurvedic practice remain the main reason behind its support. People who have tried and tested the method reveal that oil pulling should not be used with the intention of reversing severe cases such as tooth decay. However, it is indeed a great way to support supplemental therapy.

People tried the method after recommendations were made and almost all of them supported one benefit or the other. While some experimenters claimed it worked wonders in whitening their teeth the natural way, others believed it helped them get rid of the bad breath in no time.

Reported Benefits of Traditional Ayurvedic Practice

An article published on the Earth Clinic website, the practice of oil pulling is reported to be associated with a lot of health benefits. Oil pulling is said to cure: gum and mouth diseases, allergies, stiff joints, high blood pressure, asthma, migraines, constipation, eczema, bronchitis, lung diseases, heart diseases, arthritis, leukemia, insomnia, meningitis, cancer, menopause, varicose veins, chronic infections, AIDS, diabetes, cracked heels, and polio.

In fact, according to Dr. Karach, there are more benefits associated with oil pulling. According to him, this magical ayurvedic oil-therapy heals all types of headaches, tooth pain, bronchitis, eczema, thrombosis, ulcers, kidney and heart diseases, intestinal diseases, woman's diseases and encephalitis. Preventively, oil pulling is also considered beneficial in the healing and curing of malignant tumors. Paralysis, chronic blood diseases, diseases of stomach, nerves, liver and lungs, and sleeplessness can also be cured by regularly following the oil pulling process.

Now if you check the list above, it definitely appears to be very impressive. And interestingly, there could be a lot of truth in it. In fact, the majority of the benefits associated with oil pulling are actually, indirectly linked with one benefit —eliminating gum and mouth diseases.

Here's more data on this:

- *Oil pulling completely eliminates bacteria:* According to a study published in the year 2008, the method of oil pulling using sesame oil lead to a great reduction in the

Streptococcus Mutans present in the plaque. The method is said to be so effective, that the significant reduction can be experienced in as little as 2-week time. Not to forget, the reduction in streptococcus mutans is extremely beneficial for the health of your mouth because it is the primary reason of tooth decay and plaque.

- *It reduces gingivitis and plaque:* This was the study that revealed the importance of using oil pulling method for reducing gingivitis and plaque and compared the method with using chlorhexidine mouthwash, which is known to be loaded with various harmful chemicals. Now knowing the benefits of both the methods are almost same with oil pulling offering no side effects, which option would you like to go with? Oil pulling, of course!

- *Improves bad breath:* The most obvious result of using oil pulling method for health benefits includes improvement in bad, stinky breath. Most of the times, the main cause behind bad breath is the presence of bacteria in the mouth. When the amount of bacteria is reduced in the mouth, bad breath is naturally cured.

Claimed Benefits beyond Mouth?

As far as oral benefits are concerned, oil pulling is considered great for your oral health including:

1. Prevention of mouth and gum diseases, such as gingivitis and cavities
2. Overall strengthening of jaws, gums, and teeth.
3. Prevention of throat dryness, mouth dryness, and lip discoloration
4. Prevention for bad breath
5. Potential natural remedy to treat weak, bleeding gums
6. Possible natural remedy for general soreness and TMJ in the jaw area

According to ancient health practitioners associated with ayurvedic studies, oil pulling can significantly reduce more than just diseases of the throat and mouth. Nowadays, a number of holistic health practitioners around the world have adopted this oral health treatment method for various health concerns.

The following is the list of benefits of oil pulling for your overall health:

1. Relief from migraine headaches
2. Correcting the imbalances in hormone
3. Reducing arthritis inflammation
4. Helps in reducing the effects of eczema
5. Aids in gastro-enteritis
6. Aids in reducing the symptoms of bronchitis
7. People even claim improved vision benefits
8. Helps in reducing sinus congestion
9. Reduce hangover after the consumption of alcohol
10. Helps reducing pain

11. Helps in the detoxification of the body of harmful organisms and metals
12. Control allergic symptoms

In short, the benefits of oil pulling does not only stick to your mouth or oral health, the claims are much beyond that and are associated with your overall health and well being.

How Do You Do Oil Pulling?

While many people still use sesame oil for oil pulling, it is highly recommended that you use coconut oil for the procedure since coconut oil itself possesses various health benefits. Most of these benefits are discussed later in the book. Also, swishing coconut oil is a better option as compared to sunflower or sesame oil due to the difference in the taste.

This is what you need to do:

Step 1: Put one tablespoon of coconut oil in your mouth.

Step 2: Start swishing around the coconut oil in your mouth. The best way to do is to keep yourself busy with some other activity as you continue swishing oil in your mouth. You can do while doing the dishes, cooking or any other household activity that keeps you engaged. However, in a perfect world you would be expected to curl up your body in a meditation pose while putting all your energy in focusing on the swishing procedure. Continue the oil swishing procedure for 15-20 minutes (you may not be able to hold it up for that long in the first few days, but keep practicing until you can make it up to 20 minutes straights). Just focus and make sure the oil is traveling all around your mouth as you pull the oil and swish it.

Step 3: When you are done swishing the oil, spit out the pulled oil in the basin or toilet. The oil will transform into some watery, milky substance. This will ensure that you have successfully pulled oil during the procedure and you did it for sufficient time. Also, your mouth should not be oily after the procedure. If you find it oily or if you feel traces of oil in you mouth, then you may not have been completely successful in your attempt. You did not pull the oil long enough and you might have to give it another go.

Step 4: Prepare lukewarm water and add sea salt in it. Now rinse your mouth with this salty water thoroughly and follow up cleaning your mouth with a mouthwash or brush your teeth.

Some important things to remember:

- Regardless of which oil you are choosing for oil pulling, only use unrefined, cold-pressed oil.
- Oil pulling procedure should ideally be performed first thing in the morning, i.e. only on an empty stomach.
- It is essential that you rinse your mouth and brush your teeth immediately after oil pulling.
- It is highly recommended to spit out the pulled oil in the toilet because the bacteria in your mouth can be full of harmful germs. Thus, avoid spitting in the sink.
- Since the pulled oil is loaded with extremely toxic pathogens, never swallow the oil. Spit it in the toilet immediately after the procedure is complete.
- It is best to rinse your mouth after spitting the oil with lukewarm, salty water. Use only sea salt.
- Clean your toothbrush thoroughly after brushing your teeth. Next time, use only when it is completely dried up.

- It is also recommended to use different oil for practicing the procedure, including coconut oil, sesame oil, and sunflower oil.
- If you can dedicate time to oil pulling, it is best to calmly sit down and do it with focus to be successful in your first attempt.

This is it! An extremely effective, affordable, and simple way to help the natural detoxification system of your body to operate at its best! While you may not be blessed with super powers even after regular practicing of oil pulling procedure, you will definitely experience various health benefits and a bright smile for sure!

Why You Should Start Oil Pulling Today

In addition to the benefits already stated, there are many other reasons why oil pulling is highly beneficial in eliminating bacteria in your mouth and gum pockets. These are stated below.

Things You Need to Know

1. Most natural oils are already well known for the anti-bacterial properties they posses. There are studies conducted on both sunflower seed oil and sesame oil that demonstrates their ability to fight bacteria and eliminate it. Moreover, some oils (including sesame oil) also have anti-inflammatory properties.
2. It is important to remember that the time set for oil pulling, which is 20 minutes, is essential. This is a condition that should be followed under all circumstances because in this time the oil can thoroughly seep into your mouth and gum pockets. As

far as brushing your teeth or using a mouthwash for oral health is concerned, both these practices last only a few minutes. However, the prolonged time for the oil pulling procedure ensures that the natural anti-bacterial agent remains in your mouth for longer and works effectively in killing the bacteria. Using this method for at least 20 minutes ensures you that it reaches the harmful bacteria hiding inside your mouth and keeps your pockets protected.

3. Of course, oil is – as we all know – oily! When you are swishing it in your mouth, it will do what oil does. Unlike brushing your teeth, in which the toothpaste only reaches the areas where it is brushed, oil when swished around your mouth seeps onto the nooks and crannies of your mouth and gums.

4. For 20 minutes, you are expected to swish the oil aggressively around your mouth, pushing and swishing it back and forth across your mouth and gums. This will help you press down the naturally beneficial oil into the pockets of your gums. Again, making sure you do it for 20 minutes will help the oil go deeper into the pockets and eliminate bacteria completely.

As we practice oil pulling on a regular basis, we should observe if it is really making a difference and actually killing the bacteria as it claims. Our personal observation is what will satisfy us and answer our questions although there are various studies that support this contention.

Introduction to Common Oils Used for Oil Pulling

The taste and texture of the oil used for oil pulling are the first few factors that people take into account before deciding which one to use. While there are options including coconut oil, sesame seed oil, sunflower seed oil, and even some tree oils, it is best to consider the benefits each one holds before deciding which one to use for oil pulling.

What Oils Can I Use?

The information we share here will help you decide which oil is best for oil pulling procedure. Keep reading!

Sesame oil

Sesame oil, also known as the 'queen of oils' is associated with various health benefits. In fact, the ayurvedic procedure of oil pulling started with using sesame seed oil. Why? Not only does the oil have anti-bacterial and anti-inflammatory properties, there are other various benefits associated with sesame seed oil that are believed to be helpful to achieve all the remaining health benefits of oil pulling.

But is that really true? Read on to find out.

Natural sesame oil is not a modern choice. In fact, the oil has been used as an effective healing medicine for thousands of years. According to Vedas, the oil is known to have excellent health benefits for humans. It possesses natural antibacterial properties to treat common skin pathogens, including streptococcus and staphylococcus. Other than that, it also treats skin fungi effectively. Not only is sesame seed oil an anti-inflammatory agent; it is also a natural antiviral.

As far as oral health is concerned, an experiment conducted by the students of Maharishi International College in Fairfield, Iowa, revealed that with regular use of sesame oil for rinsing their mouth (oil pulling), it resulted in an 85 percent reduction in the bacteria that caused gingivitis.

However, due to the foul taste of the oil, it was difficult to hold and swish it around the mouth for 20 minutes. Also, with more oil options, people tend to switch to oils that offered more or better benefits and were easier to hold in the mouth.

Sesame seed oil, despite of all the other reasons, remain the most widely used oil for oil pulling procedure.

Sunflower Oil

Next that comes in line is the sunflower oil. A long list of benefits is associated with the usage of sunflower oil that keeps your body strong and healthy. Unfortunately, a number of people are not aware of these benefits and thus ignore the importance of using this amazing oil for their health.

As far as oil pulling with sunflower oil is concerned, it is pretty much similar to sesame oil, with natural antibacterial and anti-inflammatory properties. However, there are other health benefits listed below:

1. Sunflower seed can improve heart health
2. It is a natural energy booster
3. It lowers the risk of cardiovascular diseases and reduces the chance of heart attack
4. Lowers risk of developing infant infections
5. Sunflower oil is a natural antioxidant
6. Prevents arthritis
7. Natural moisturizer

8. Prevents colon cancer and asthma

With that impressive list of health benefits, sunflower seed oil is definitely a go for oil pulling. However, the benefits are assumed to be limited as the oil is only used for swishing. In any case, with so many health benefits associated with the regular use of this oil, sunflower oil is recommended oil for oil pulling.

Grapeseed Oil

Like the name suggests, grapeseed oil is extracted from grape seeds, typically wine grapes. While these seeds are usually discarded during the wine making process, they soon become the most efficient and profitable sideline.

Today, grapeseed oil is widely used for two main purposes: culinary and cosmetic application. Why? The benefits of using grapeseed oil in food and as a cosmetic are never-ending. This affordable oil is light in both flavor and color, with a slight hint of nuttiness. The popular beneficial compound it contains is called linoleic acid.

Even during the ayurvedic practice, grapeseed oil was a popular choice. Today, considering the health benefits of this oil, it is widely used for oil pulling purposes. The best part is that grapeseed oil is an excellent source of vitamin E and essential fatty acids. The flavonoids and polyphenols present in this oil are loaded with powerful antioxidant compounds. These are the main nutrients because of which grapeseed oil is considered healthy.

In addition to these, grapeseed oil has the following benefits because of which it becomes one of the most widely used oil for oil pulling procedure:

1. The flavonoid present in the grapeseed oil is an unbelievably powerful antioxidant, about 50 times stronger than vitamin E and C. This offer better protection against tissue and cellular damage by free radicals.
2. The oil is perfect for boosting your heart and cardiovascular health by controlling and balancing LDL bad cholesterol level. At the same time, it has the qualities to increase HDL cholesterol levels, which is known to be good cholesterol. Eventually, the risk of developing coronary diseases is reduced.
3. Loaded with linoleic acid, it can offer great health benefits to people with diabetes.
4. Grapeseed oil can also repair and strengthen broken or damaged blood vessels and capillaries.
5. This oil is rich in minerals, vitamins and has great moisturizing properties.

Keeping all those benefits in mind, grapeseed oil, which is also commonly used for cooking, is great for oil pulling practice.

Olive Oil

Olive oil is another significant choice among other oils for oil pulling. Without a doubt, olive oil, especially in its extra-virgin form, is one of the best oils on earth. Olive oil is one of the primary choices of people practicing the oil pulling ayurvedic practice today because this oil has proved to be effective against various diseases.

Some of these include:

Cancer

The phytonutrient present in olive oil behaves exactly like ibuprofen for reducing the effects of inflammation. This helps decrease the risk of breast cancer.

Heart Diseases

Olive oil can effectively lower the overall blood cholesterol, triglycerides, and LDL-cholesterol. On the other hand, it does not affect the HDL cholesterol levels. This in turn controls the fatty patches formation and saves you from falling victim to a number of heart diseases.

Blood Pressure

According to recent studies, regular consumption of this magic oil can help reduce both diastolic and systolic blood pressure.

Oxidative Stress

Loaded with antioxidants, olive oil is especially rich in vitamin E. This helps you minimize the risk of developing cancer and its re-occurrence.

Obesity

One of the main reasons this oil is used for culinary purpose is to treat obesity. Although olive oil is high in calories, it has shown great results in reducing the levels of obesity on the record.

Other than these, olive oil has also shown great benefits in reducing the risk for diabetes, osteoporosis, and rheumatoid arthritis. Most of the benefits listed here are similar to the benefits of oil pulling. Strange right? The health benefits offered by certain oils are somewhere linked to the benefits of the overall results of oil pulling. This is because the entire practice involves swishing and holding these oils in the mouth. Moreover, since olive oil is widely used for cooking, it is easier to hold this edible oil in the mouth for long.

All these factors make olive oil one of the best oils to use for oil pulling.

Coconut Oil

In comparison to sunflower oil, sesame oil and grapeseed oil, coconut oil is the most popular oil to be used for oil pulling. Traditionally, when the procedure of oil pulling was introduced, Indians used different oils for oil pulling – including sunflower and sesame oil.

While oil pulling can be used with pretty much any edible oil, coconut oil is usually a preference these days because of the health benefits it possesses. Why? Because it is one of the few foods that are actually classified as 'superfoods. 'Coconut oil is beneficial since it is a unique combination of healthy fatty acids that has profound health effects. These include efficient brain function, fat loss and others among the rest. For better understanding, here's a list of health benefits of coconut oil:

1. Coconut oil is known for its health benefits since it contains a unique combination of healthy fatty acids that are loaded with effective medicinal properties.
2. In order to obtain maximum health benefits, most people use coconut oil for cooking.
3. The healthy ingredient is effective in burning fat since it naturally boosts your energy expenditure.
4. As far as using coconut oil for oil pulling is concerned, it is considered amazing oil because of the lauric acid present in it. Lauric acid can kill bacteria, fungi, and viruses. Using it for oral health can be greatly beneficial.
5. Various health issues are linked to seizures and fatty acids present in coconut oil are turned into ketones, which naturally reduce seizures.

Other than these health benefits, it is easier to hold this oil in the mouth because of its acceptable taste. Since it is crucial to hold and swish the oil in the mouth for at least 20 minutes, oil pulling using coconut oil is a preferred way.

Indeed, coconut oil – because of the endless health and oral benefits – is also recommended for practicing oil pulling.

Final Word

While the procedure of oil pulling belongs to a different era, the comeback and popularity of this method itself proves that there is reality associated to it with reference to health benefits. The modern day practice of oil pulling further justifies the usage of this method to benefit from various health benefits it has to offer.

With the information shared in this book, you are all ready to try this method out yourself. In fact, if you were a little skeptical about the concept of oil pulling before reading this book, I believe after reading all the health benefits of this method, you will be more than prepared to give it a try and gain from the oral and health benefits associated with oil pulling.

Get started today because your optimal health is just one step away!

Good luck!